Pregnancy Associated

Exposures

&

the Outcome of ADHD:

A Review

By: Michanna Talley, JD, MS, BS, Cert.

Published by Jazi Gifts by Michanna, LLC, Publishing Division

Greenville, South Carolina

www.jazigifts.com

1-888-778-4808.

ISBN 978-0-9842684-1-2

Pregnancy Associated Exposures & The Outcome of ADHD: A Review

By: Michanna Talley, JD, MS, BS, Cert.

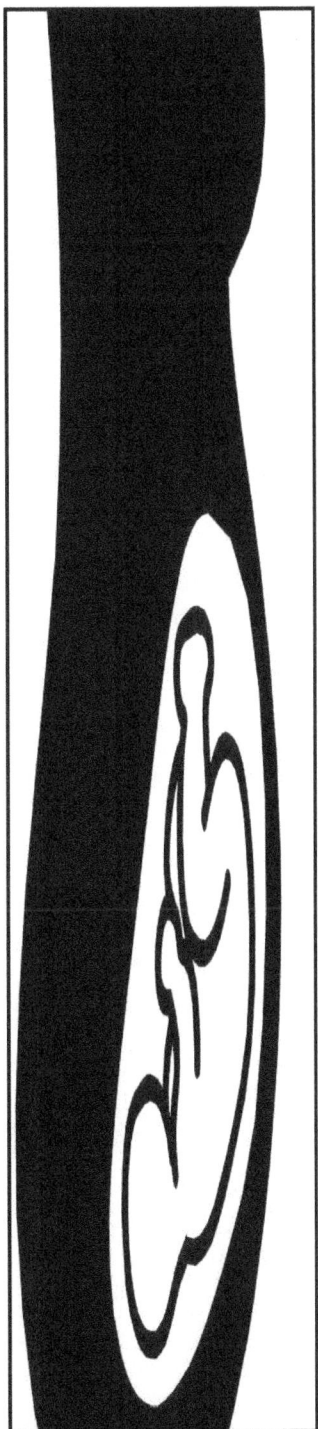

Other Titles by Michanna Talley:

7 Steps to Healthy Natural Hair

Views of Falls Park

The Effect of Land Use on Biodiversity

TABLE OF CONTENTS

Prologue 11

Introduction 13

Methods 15

Exposures 17

    1. Genetic Predisposition & Smoking 19

    2. Environmental Toxicants 25

    3. Low Birth Weight 29

    4. Alcohol Consumption 31

    5. Coffee Consumption 33

    6. Stress 35

Discussion 37

Conclusion 43

References 45

About the Author 47

PROLOGUE

In our present day society, Attention Deficit Hyperactivity Disorder (ADHD) has a seemingly increased presence in adolescents and adults. This review seeks to address possible causes of ADHD to increase understanding into the disorder. This review also seeks to satisfy the curiosity of the author of this review, who, with a personally short attention span, sought to obtain information regarding ADHD, finding that the majority of the symptoms of the disorder are personally met. An additional step was also taken by completing an online test which produced the results of "moderately ADHD," which is one step below "severely ADHD." This result was only due to the honest answering of questions including personal changes that have been imposed on oneself to overcome symptoms which are present, yet are purposefully suppressed. Through completion of this review, a great amount of information and knowledge was gained.

INTRODUCTION

Attention Deficit Hyperactivity Disorder (ADHD) is one of the most commonly diagnosed behavioral disorders. It is illustrated primarily by short attention spans, the inability to concentrate, and increased hyperactivity and impulsivity. These symptoms are primarily those of the external version of the disorder, while an internal version of the disorder also exists. If medically diagnosed, medical treatment is available which seeks to reverse or nullify the recognized symptoms mentioned previously. The causes of ADHD have not been pinned down definitively, but there are many prenatal factors to be weighed. These factors include genetic predisposition, smoking, alcohol use, caffeine consumption, and the presence of stress during pregnancy. Postnatal factors such as a non-favorable family environment may possibly increase symptoms and their severity. A favorable family environment may decrease symptoms, causing them to disappear completely or possibly create in the child an ability to manage the symptoms. As this is a review of pregnancy-associated exposures, post-natal factors will not be discussed further.

METHODS

PubMed, a service of the US National Library of Medicine and the National Institutes of Health, was searched to obtain articles about pregnancy and ADHD. The following keywords were used: pregnancy-associated exposures and ADHD, prenatal and ADHD, and pregnancy and ADHD. Results were further limited by full text access availability and language. Similar papers to those chosen during the process were also obtained. Studies which directly address various prenatal factors and ADHD specifically were selected. Ten articles which included relevant exposure and outcome variables were chosen. The ten selected articles describe several studies with various prenatal factors addressed. Studies include those carried out in and outside of the United States. Articles will be presented based on the prenatal factors addressed in the article (several articles tackle more than one factor).

EXPOSURES

GENETIC PREDISPOSITION & SMOKING

A prospective longitudinal study, a study in which repeated observations are carried out over long periods of time, was conducted out to determine if an interaction was present between the dopamine transporter genotype (DAT1 – studied previously in regards to disorders such as ADHD, Parkinson's, alcoholism, and schizophrenia[4]) along with smoking to ADHD symptoms. Over a 15 year period, 305 participants (initially infants) in the study were assessed. Controls (baseline groups) were used to deal with confounding (variables affecting the outcome of the study) and participants who were handicapped, dropped out of the study, and/or did not participate in blood sampling were excluded. Information regarding ADHD symptoms was obtained through diagnostic interviews completed by parents and the participants themselves. From these interviews, the presence of maternal smoking was ascertained. Blood samples were taken from participants to isolate DNA to determine the presence or absence of the DAT1 genotype. With the obtained information, bivariate statistical analyses (analysis of the relationship between two variables) were carried out and adjustments were made for confounding variables. No significance was found between ADHD symptoms and the DAT1 genotype, however males who were exposed to prenatal smoke and were positive for the DAT1 gene, were found to have significantly higher hyperactive-impulsive scores. This finding was true overall and is consistent with like studies previously completed[2].

Another study was carried out using twins between the ages of seven and eighteen as participants (747 families and 183 control families). If one or both twins were deceased, autistic, or mentally retarded, the families were excluded from the study. Parent interviews using questionnaires were conducted to obtain information regarding the attention and hyperactivity of the children as well as their own conduct during pregnancy (smoking, alcohol use, familial conduct, etc.). DNA samples were also taken. Six subtypes of ADHD were analyzed using multivariate regression models (a technique used to model and analyze several variables) based on the Diagnostic and Statistical Manual of Mental Disorders (DSM-IV). Adjustments for the sex of the twins were made so as to prevent confounding. Significantly higher ADHD scores were obtained in those who were exposed to prenatal smoking. Additionally, the risk of ADHD was found to be higher for children who were exposed to prenatal smoking and had the presence of the DAT1 440 gene or the DRD4 gene (examined in relation to neuropsychiatric disorders and variation from normal behavior[11]). However, there was no significance found between the ADHD phenotype, prenatal smoking exposure, and the DAT1 480 gene[9].

The DRD4 gene was also targeted in another study. This study also looked at the presence of the allele coupled with prenatal smoke exposure to the presence of ADHD. Included in the study were 539 subjects between the ages of five and seventeen years old who were clinically diagnosed with a combined subtype of ADHD (based on DSM-IV) and had a parent and at least one full unaffected sibling available for DNA collection (407 total). Children who were autistic, epileptic, had learning difficulties, had brain disorders, has any disorder with symptoms that may mimic that of ADHD, and/or with IQ's lower than 70, were excluded from the study. Mothers of the children provided prenatal information using questionnaires. Information regarding ADHD symptoms of the children was obtained from both parent and teacher feedback. Various models and variables were used to prevent possible confounding or bias (example: adding dummy variables). A significant effect was found between the parents' scores of participants regarding ADHD symptoms and the presence of the targeted gene while a significant effect was found between the teachers' scores of participants and the exposure to prenatal smoking. Conclusively, no significant effect was found between the presence of the DRD4 gene with smoking exposure and ADHD status[1].

ENVIRONMENTAL TOXICANTS

Continuing with the exposure to smoking, a study was done to determine if prenatal smoking exposure coupled with prenatal lead exposure had an effect on the outcome of ADHD. Data was obtained from a cross-sectional household survey, a survey used to observe a subset of a population. The outcome of ADHD was based on a medical diagnosis in addition to medication use. Children who had a medical diagnosis but were not on medication and vice versa were excluded from the study. Prenatal smoking exposure information was obtained from the parents' reports. The presence of a metabolite of nicotine in the children's serum was also used, but used secondarily. Lead concentration was measured in blood samples of the 135 participants by spectrophotometry (measuring the wavelength of light). Several confounding variables were identified and examined (age, sex, race, birth weight, etc.). Using multivariate analysis, prenatal exposure to smoking and lead were found to be significant predictors of ADHD. Further, the amount of lead exposure alone was also found to be significant[3].

Hexachlorobenzene (HCB) is a chemical used in agriculture and industrial processes. It is possible to be ingested or inhaled by humans due to its use as a fungicide on crops. A study was completed to study the prenatal exposure of HCB on social behavior, including ADHD. In this cohort study (study carried out on a group of people that share a common characteristic within a set period), participants were children born at the hospital at which this study took place. All participants were four years of age and information was available regarding their organochlorine compound (OC) levels at birth (HCB is an OC). Scores regarding social behavior and the presence or absence of ADHD symptoms were obtained using information obtained from each child's teacher. Information was also obtained regarding several possible confounding variables (gender, alcohol exposure, diet, breast-feeding, etc.) two years following the birth of each child. Adjustment was made for these variables by using multivariate models. The presence of ADHD was defined as having six or more symptoms of either inattention and/or hyperactivity-impulsivity based on the DSM-IV. HCB concentrations were further divided into four categories (<0.5, 0.5-0.99, 1.00-1.49, and >1.5 ng/mL). The study was conducted on two separate groups of participants (471 total). HCB concentrations greater than 1.5 ng/mL were found to associate with inattention and hyperactivity. However, in one study group these results were found to be significant, while in another study group they were not found to be statistically significant[10].

Another cohort study was used to determine the effect, if any, that tetrachloroethylene (PCE) has on ADHD. PCE is found in contaminated drinking water. This may be due to the water source or the type of pipes through which the water flows (example: vinyl-lined asbestos-cement (VL/AC) pipes). Children born in areas with VL/AC pipes between 1969 and 1983 were included in the study. A total of 1910 exposed children were compared to 1927 unexposed children. They were matched up based on their month and year of birth. Information regarding water sources, residential history, behavioral disorders, and possible confounders, were obtained through questionnaires. Due to a medical diagnosis, 404 children were defined as having ADHD. Children with several confounding variables (multiple birth, lead poisoning, mental retardation, marijuana use, etc.) were excluded from the study. There was no significant finding of an increased risk of ADHD with the exposure of PCE using multivariate analysis[6].

LOW BIRTH WEIGHT

A cohort study was also completed regarding low birth weight and ADHD. Infants born between 24 to 36 weeks gestation with birth weights between 1.32 and 3.31 pounds were compared to infants born between 37 to 43 weeks gestation with birth weights between 5.64 and 10.87 pounds. Parents completed surveys regarding symptoms of ADHD and abuse of various substances. Mothers also provided information through self-report, producing possible confounding variables. Participants who did not complete the questionnaire, attended school to address developmental problems, had neurosensory impairment, or were severely depressed, were excluded from the study. Adjustments were made to control confounding variables when possible. A total of 162 participants with very low birth weight (VLBW) were split into two groups: those who were small for gestational age (SGA) due to growth retardation (52 participants) and those with a birth weight that was appropriate for gestational age (AGA), but were born premature (110 participants). After using SPSS (a statistical software commonly used in the field of Public Health) for statistical analysis, a relationship was found to exist between VLBW individuals and ADHD. Also, it was determined that SGA is a better predictor of future ADHD symptoms than AGA[12].

ALCOHOL CONSUMPTION

In the previously mentioned studies, one of the possible confounding variables is that of alcohol consumption during pregnancy. Information for this retrospective study, a study that looks backwards in time, was obtained from twin mothers by way of a telephone interview survey. The ADHD diagnosis of the 922 children was based on maternal report. Those children with six or more symptoms of ADHD (based on the DSM-IV) which were present prior to the age of seven were included in the study. Information regarding prenatal alcohol consumption was used to create five categories (1-10 days of <5 drinks/day, 11-35 days of <5 drinks/day, >35 days of <5 drinks/day, 1-10 days of ≥5 drinks/day, and having ≥5 drinks/day in 11+ days). Information regarding smoking, a possible confounder, was also obtained, categorized (never smoked, regular smoker but not during pregnancy, smoking during 1st trimester only, smoked 1-15 cigarettes/day beyond the 1st trimester, and 16+ cigarettes/day beyond the first trimester), and then controlled. Although an association between increased ADHD risk and alcohol abuse was found, it was not deemed to be significant[7].

COFFEE CONSUMPTION

A prospective cohort study was completed to determine if an association was present between coffee consumption during pregnancy and ADHD. Information for the study was obtained through two self administered questionnaires. One questionnaire allowed for information regarding coffee consumption to be obtained, while the other was in reference to confounding variables (smoking, alcohol, etc.). Coffee consumption was categorized as follows: 0, 1-3, 4-9, and 10+ cups of coffee a day. Additional information of the consumption of other sources of caffeine such as tea and chocolate were also obtained. The presence of ADHD symptoms was based on information in hospital files. A total of 74 participants between the ages of three and twelve had at least six out of a possible nine symptoms based on the DSM-IV. Children with diagnoses of autism, mental retardation, and developmental disorders were excluded from the study. Adjustments were made for varying follow up times and possible confounding variables. It was found that intrauterine exposure to coffee consumption of ten or more cups a day leads to an increased risk of ADHD. However, this finding became statistically insignificant after adjustments for confounding variables were made. Results did not change when several types of adjustments were made for various possible confounding variables[8].

STRESS

The last reviewed study sought to determine if an association between maternal prenatal stress and ADHD exists. Included in the study were 203 participants who were between the ages of six and twelve. Participants were targeted by way of the hospital's specialized care facility. ADHD determinations were based on diagnoses following clinical evaluations in addition to interviews with parents and teachers, and information obtained from school reports. Children with developmental disorders, Tourette syndrome, or other medical conditions that could possibly affect their participation in the program were excluded from the study. The presence or absence of stress was obtained through interviews of mothers using a questionnaire. Their prenatal stress levels were then categorized based on level and the trimester at which they were experienced (scored 1 to 5, with 5 being the highest). The severity of ADHD symptoms was compared to the severity of stress using ANOVA (an analysis of variance where it is determined whether or not significant differences exist). It was found that increased stress caused more severe ADHD symptoms. The later the stress occurred (example: occurring in the third trimester), the more severe the ADHD symptoms were found to be[5].

DISCUSSION

Several of the studied factors were found to lead to an increase in ADHD symptoms. Very low birth weight, prenatal stress, and prenatal lead exposure coupled with smoking all led to an increased presence of ADHD. Other factors were also found to have the same outcome, however, at times these results were significant and at other times they were not. Both prenatal alcohol and coffee consumption were found to lead to an increase in ADHD symptoms, but not significantly. Out of the three reviewed studies regarding genetics and prenatal smoking exposure, the association with the outcome of ADHD in one of the studies was found to be significant and found to be insignificant in the remaining two studies. This also proved true for the presence of the environmental toxin HCB. It was initially found to have a significant impact on the outcome of ADHD, but became insignificant after adjustments for confounding variables were made. These results are somewhat unstable and therefore there are obvious limitations of these studies.

Within the various studies, the way in which ADHD was diagnosed varied. For example, in Strang-Karlsson et al. the determination of ADHD was based on a questionnaire, while in Braun et al. the determination of ADHD was based on parent report of medical diagnosis and stimulant medication use[12,3]. In other studies, the determination was based on self-report by participants (adolescents), record of symptoms in hospital records, and/or teacher provided information. Also, a lot of this questioning, including questioning regarding prenatal activity, was done retrospectively. This requires that interviewees be honest and remember correctly. It is possible that only one or neither of these requirements are met by those completing the questionnaire. Even if the questionnaires are answered honestly and correctly, there are many other variables that may explain the observed outcomes. In addition to this, there is also a problem of non-response. This provides little to no information to those conducting the study and can lead to the exclusion of participants. A relatively high rate of non-response (as in Ribas-Fitó et al.[10]) could possibly change the findings of the study.

In some studies, possible confounding variables are not addressed at all, as in Knopik et al[7]. In this study, other possible confounding factors not examined (family adversity, traumatic brain injury, marital problems, and ADHD symptoms in the parents and/or other family members) were mentioned. This is further illustrated by the study completed by Grizenko et al[5]. Although this study focused on the presence of prenatal stress on the outcome of ADHD, the following factors were mentioned as having a possible effect on results: mothers who seek help for stress and are therefore better able to deal with it as well as the postnatal environment of the child. These variables amongst others may lead to an under or over estimation of the outcome of ADHD, with which genetic variations may or may not have an effect. The problem of underestimation due to bias was specifically referenced in Linnet et al[8].

The issue of sample size was also found to be a limitation in several studies. In both Neuman et al. and Linnet et al. this was revealed[9,8]. Separate from sample size, the issue of lack of ethnic diversity was present in Becker et al[2]. The lack of diversity creates the problem of the results not being generalizable (capable of being applied to society as a whole). However, in some studies strengths were present.

In at least one of the reviewed studies, a large sample size was present, therefore adding increased reliability to the study. Also, even though some studies did not, other studies did identify confounders, took them into account, and then adjusted for their presence. In other studies such as Janulewicz et al., little confounding was found in regards to the presence of other water contaminants[6]. Another

strength present in several of the studies was the use of exposure and

outcome scales and/or categories. This allowed for severity of either

the exposure or the outcome to be weighed, or possibly both. For

example, in Altink et al. ADHD symptoms were categorized into total,

hyperactive, inattentive, and oppositional groups[1]. In total, several

different variables were taken into account in regards to ADHD.

Putting all these variables together may increase information regarding

pregnancy exposures and the outcome of ADHD.

CONCLUSION

The information available in regards to exposures and outcomes of ADHD is rather vast. However, due to the additive nature of these exposures, pinpointing direct causes of any disorder, including ADHD can be difficult. All genetic and environmental factors must be studied in future research to further understand this common disorder. On the other hand one must be certain to also take into account the postnatal environment of individuals that can possibly prove stronger than the prenatal exposures that may lead to the presence of symptoms of ADHD. Nevertheless, negative prenatal and postnatal behavior should be erased or at least limited. This can begin to be instituted through prevention programs organized by clinical and public health organizations.

REFERENCES

1. Altink, M.E., Arias-Vásquez, A., Franke, B., Slaats-Willemse, D.I.E., Buschgens, C.J.M., et al. (2008). The Dopamine Receptor D4 7-Repeat Allele and Prenatal Smoking in ADHD-Affected Children and Their Unaffected Siblings: No Gene-Environment Interaction. *Journal of Child Psychology and Psychiatry*, 49:10, 1053-1060.

2. Becker, K., El-Faddagh, M., Schmidt, M.H., Esser, G., & Laught, M. (2008). Interaction of Dopamine Transporter Genotype with Prenatal Smoke Exposure on ADHD Symptoms. *The Journal of Pediatrics*, 152, 263-269.

3. Braun, J.M., Kahn, R.S., Froehlich, T., Auinger, P., & Lanphear, B.P. (2006). Exposures to Environmental Toxicants and Attention Deficit Hyperactivity Disorder in U.S. Children. *Environmental Health Perspectives*, 114, 1904-1909.

4. Fuke, S., Suo S., Takahashi, N., Koike, H., Sasagawa, N., et al. (2001). The VNTR Polymorphism of the Human Dopamine transporter (DAT1) Gene Affects Gene Expression. *The Pharmacogenomics Journal*, 1, 152-156.

5. Grizenko, N., Shayan, Y.R., Polotskaia, A., Ter-Stepanian, M., & Joober, R. (2008). Relation of Maternal Stress During Pregnancy to Symptom Severity and Response to Treatment in Children with ADHD. *Journal of Psychiatry & Neuroscience*, 33, 10-16.

6. Janulewicz, P.A., White, R.F., Winter, M.R., Weinberg, J.M., Gallagher, L.E., et al. (2008). Risk of Learning and Behavioral Disorders Following Prenatal and Early Postnatal Exposure to Tetrachloroethylene (PCE)-Contaminated Drinking Water. *Neurotoxicology and Teratology*, 30, 175-185.

7. Knopik, V.S., Heath, A.C., Jacob, T., Slutske, W.S., Bucholz, K.K., et al. (2006). Maternal Alcohol Use Disorder and Offspring ADHD: Disentangling Genetic and Environmental Effects Using a Children-of-Twins Design. *Psychological Medicine*, 36, 1461-1471.

8. Linnet, K.M., Wisborg, K., Secher, N.J., Thomsen, P.H., Obel, C., et al. (2008). Coffee Consumption During Pregnancy and the Risk of Hyperkinetic Disorder and ADHD: A Prospective Cohort Study. *Acta Paediatrica*, 98, 173-179.

9. Neuman, R.J., Lobos, E., Reich, W., Henderson, C.A., Sun, L., & Todd, R.D. (2007). Prenatal Smoking Exposure and Dopaminergic Genotypes Interact to Cause a Severe ADHD Subtype. *Biological Psychiatry*, 61, 1320-1328.

10. Ribas-Fitó, N., Torrent, M., Carrizo, D., Júlvez, J., Grimalt, J.O., & Sunyer, J. (2007). Exposure to Hexachlorobenzene During Pregnancy and Children's Social Behavior at 4 Years of Age. *Environmental Health Perspectives*, 115:3, 447-450.

11. Seaman, M.I., Fisher, J.B., Chang, F., & Kidd, K.K. (1999). Tandem Duplication Polymorphism Upstream of the Dopamine D4 Receptor Gene (DRD4). *American Journal of Medical Genetics*, 88(6), 705-709.

12. Strang-Karlsson, S., Räikkönen, K., Pesonen, A., Kajantie, E., Paavonen, E.J., et al. (2008). Very Low Birth Weight and Behavioral Symptoms of Attention Deficit Hyperactivity Disorder in Young Adulthood: The Helsinki Study of Very-Low-Birth-Weight Adults. *The American Journal of Psychiatry*, 165:10 1345-1353.

ABOUT THE AUTHOR

MICHANNA TALLEY is a lawyer in Greenville, South Carolina. She is a graduate of Stetson University College of Law located in Tampa Bay, FL. Michanna also holds both a Master's and a Bachelor's degree in Biology from Howard University in Washington, DC. She also holds Graduate Certification in the field of Public Health, specifically in Epidemiology and Biostatistics from Drexel University located in Philadelphia, Pennslyvania. Prior to entering law school, Michanna was an Adjunct Instructor teaching General Biology 101 and 102 and prior to that was a Nucleic Acids Microbiologist working in the field of Biodefense in the DC metropolitan area. Even with her legal career, Michanna has continued to keep one foot in the scientific field by teaching online for University of Phoenix as well as local universities. Michanna also is able to have an outlet for her creative side with her business, Jazi Gifts (www.jazigifts.com).